Silent Inflammation

The Hidden Link to Chronic Diseases and Natural Ways to Heal

Harmony Royce

DEDICATION

This book is dedicated to everyone who has started the path to improved health, including those who are trying to understand their bodies, those who are trying to change, and those who are committed to changing their health for the better. I hope that anyone who is prepared to make the required changes to reverse silent inflammation and lead a healthier, more vibrant life will find this book to be a helpful guide and source of inspiration.

This book honors the tenacity, devotion, and steadfast commitment to self-care of the healthcare professionals who spend their careers assisting others, as well as the innumerable people who bravely face their obstacles. You have a strong road ahead of you, and this is only the beginning.

May you experience tremendous transformation, empowerment, and knowledge on your journey to health and healing.

DISCLAIMER

This book's content is meant exclusively for educational purposes and should not be interpreted as medical advice. The author and publisher disclaim all obligation for any negative effects or repercussions resulting from the use of the information provided, even if every effort has been taken to assure its correctness and dependability.

Any major changes to your food, exercise, or lifestyle should always be discussed with a certified healthcare provider, particularly if you are taking medication or have underlying medical conditions. Professional medical diagnosis or treatment cannot be replaced by the information in this book.

Individual outcomes may differ, and the techniques described in this book are intended to supplement professional care rather than to replace it. The author advises readers to consult healthcare professionals for individualized advice and make well-informed decisions depending on their particular situation.

CONTENTS

ACKNOWLEDGMENTS

I want to express my sincere appreciation to everyone who helped me along the way as I wrote this book. This effort would not have been accomplished without your support, wisdom, and commitment.

I want to start by expressing my gratitude to my family for their constant belief and support. Throughout this journey, your unwavering love and support have been a source of strength.

I also want to sincerely thank the medical professionals and wellness, nutrition, and inflammation specialists who have so kindly offered their knowledge and experience. The content of this book has been greatly influenced by your inputs.

To my mentors, friends, and coworkers—your comments, counsel, and careful deliberations have been invaluable in helping me hone my concepts and maintain my perspective on the wider picture. I appreciate your advice and motivation.

Last but not least, I would want to thank the readers, whose excitement and comments have demonstrated that the quest for greater knowledge and health is a continuous process. I hope that this book will be a useful tool for you as you go toward recovery and wellbeing.

With appreciation.

CHAPTER 1

COMPREHENDING INFLAMMATION WITHOUT SOUND

1.1 Inflammation: What Is It?

Acute versus Chronic Inflammation Definition

The body's natural reaction to damage, infection, or negative stimuli is inflammation. The immune system is triggered during this crucial step in order to eradicate dangers and promote recovery. Redness, heat, swelling, pain, and loss of function are the immediate, transient symptoms of acute inflammation. When you sprain your ankle, for example, the swelling and warmth you feel are signs that acute inflammation is working.

Conversely, chronic inflammation is a protracted condition in which the immune system stays engaged for weeks, months, or even years. Chronic inflammation persists and can harm tissues and organs, resulting in long-term health difficulties, in contrast to acute inflammation, which goes away after the threat has been eliminated.

The Natural Defense System of the Body

The body's first line of defense against infections, wounds, and poisons is inflammation. In order to fix damage and get rid of dangerous substances, immune cells, cytokines, and blood vessels collaborate in this process. The body's ability to isolate the issue, organize resources, and resolve it is demonstrated by acute inflammation.

On the other hand, chronic inflammation develops when the inflammatory response is miscontrolled or does not stop. Silent inflammation may result from the body unintentionally attacking its own cells and tissues as a result of this ongoing activation.

The "Silent" Nature of Inflammation

Low-grade inflammation, often known as silent inflammation, functions without the overt signs of acute inflammation. Its presence is not indicated by redness, swelling, or pain. Rather, it gradually harms tissues and organs in a covert manner. Numerous factors, including a poor diet, stress, inactivity, environmental pollutants, and even genetic predispositions, can cause this illness.

Silent inflammation frequently remains unnoticed until it presents as a chronic condition like diabetes or cardiovascular problems because it lacks obvious symptoms. It is especially harmful because of its "hidden" nature, which emphasizes the necessity of proactive health monitoring.

1.2 Inflammation's Function in the Body

The significance of the immune response

An important part of the immune system is inflammation. It is how the body delivers nutrients, hormones, and white blood cells to places that need protection or repair. When you cut your finger, for instance, inflammatory signals make sure that immune cells get there fast to stop infection and start the healing process. For survival, acute inflammation is necessary.

But this balance is upset by silent inflammation. It causes the body to experience needless wear and tear by establishing a continuous state of immunological activity that ignores an immediate threat.

Differences Between Normal Inflammatory Processes and Silent Inflammation

The normal inflammatory response is strictly controlled. They start with an alarm phase to deal with damage or infection, move on to a repair phase, and end with tissue regeneration and resolution. This resolution phase is absent in silent inflammation. Instead, a modest but persistent immune response that can damage the body's cells and tissues is maintained by low-level signals that are always circulating.

The following are some important distinctions between quiet and normal inflammation:

- **Triggering agents:** quiet inflammation is frequently caused by lifestyle choices rather than recent infections or accidents.
- Silent inflammation has no symptoms, whereas normal inflammation is visible (e.g., swelling, redness).
- **Duration:** Normal inflammation goes away as soon as the problem is resolved, whereas silent

inflammation lasts forever.

The Reasons It's Harder to Find Silent Inflammation

Because it functions beneath the surface of conventional symptoms, silent inflammation is difficult to identify. Only certain biomarkers, such as high C-reactive protein (CRP), cytokine levels, or inflammatory markers in blood tests, can be used to identify it. The significance of early detection and preventative care is highlighted by the fact that silent inflammation might worsen undetected in the absence of routine medical examinations.

1.3 Chronic Disease and Silent Inflammation

List of Disorders Associated with Silent Inflammation

Since silent inflammation has been linked to many chronic illnesses, it is an important topic for research in contemporary medicine. The following are a few ailments associated with chronic inflammation:

- Insulin resistance and type 2 diabetes can result from persistent inflammation that disrupts insulin signaling.
- **Cardiovascular Disease:** Inflammation raises the

risk of heart attacks and strokes by damaging blood vessels and causing plaque to accumulate.

- **Cancer:** By causing DNA damage and encouraging uncontrolled cell proliferation, chronic inflammation fosters an environment that is favorable to tumor formation.

- **Diseases of Neurodegeneration:** Parkinson's disease and Alzheimer's disease are linked to silent inflammation in the brain.

- **Autoimmune Conditions:** The body may attack its own tissues in an autoimmune reaction brought on by chronic inflammation.

How Prolonged Inflammation Leads to the Manifestation of Chronic Diseases

Silent inflammation frequently precedes the onset of chronic illnesses. For instance:

- Inflammatory signals in cardiovascular disease promote the buildup of plaques in arteries that are high in cholesterol. These plaques may eventually burst, leading to heart attacks or strokes.

- Chronic inflammation in adipose tissue interferes with regular metabolic processes in diabetes, resulting in insulin resistance.

- Inflammatory cytokines in the brain worsen neuronal damage in neurodegenerative illnesses, hastening cognitive decline.

These mechanisms highlight how hidden inflammation and chronic illness are intertwined.

The Financial and Individual Consequences of Ignoring Silent Inflammation

Silent inflammation has serious repercussions if ignored:

- **The financial burden:** Healthcare expenses are driven by chronic conditions associated with silent inflammation. It takes a lot of resources to treat diseases like diabetes and heart disease, requiring prescription drugs, hospital stays, and long-term care.

- **Personal Health Expenses:** Quality of life is impacted by silent inflammation. Persistent pain, cognitive deterioration, and chronic fatigue can all lower well-being and productivity.

- **Social Impact:** Chronic diseases have a cascading effect on communities, companies, and families, highlighting the collective cost of neglecting this unspoken health emergency.

People can take proactive measures to protect their health, lower their chance of developing chronic diseases, and improve their general well-being by being aware of and taking action against silent inflammation.

Recognizing the significant effects of silent inflammation on the body, its connection to chronic illnesses, and the necessity of early detection and lifestyle modification are all important aspects of understanding this hidden condition. By investigating its causes and effects, we can equip ourselves to make wise decisions for our long-term well-being.

CHAPTER 2

THE SCIENCE OF SILENT INFLAMMATION

2.1 Inflammatory Cellular Mechanisms

The Function of Inflammatory Cytokines

Small signaling proteins called inflammatory cytokines are generated by cells, especially immune cells, to mediate and control inflammation. During the immune response, they serve as messengers that help cells communicate with one another. Tumor necrosis factor-alpha (TNF-α), interleukins (IL-1, IL-6), and interferons are a few examples of inflammatory cytokines.

The body releases cytokines in response to pathogens, poisons, or injured cells in order to:

- Draw white blood cells (macrophages, neutrophils) to the site of injury.
- Encourage vasodilation to boost blood flow, which

will bring more immune cells to the injured site.

- Aid in the processes of tissue healing.

On the other hand, cytokines may be overproduced in silent or chronic inflammation, leading to a protracted immune activation. Healthy tissues and organs may sustain damage as a result of this ongoing signaling.

The Immune System's Function in Chronic Inflammation

The main functions of the immune system are tissue repair and defense against dangerous intruders. The immune response in acute inflammation is quick, focused, and ends as the threat is removed. This resolution phase is interfered with in chronic inflammation.

This is how persistent inflammation happens:

- **Persistent Threats:** The immune system may remain active due to ongoing exposure to irritants, such as toxins, infections, and poor food.

- **Autoimmune Reactions:** Sometimes the body's own tissues are mistakenly attacked by the immune system because it perceives them as danger.

- **Dysregulated Immune Response:** Even in the absence of actual danger, hyperactive immune cells continue to release inflammatory cytokines.

The immune system's incapacity to "turn off" this reaction causes silent inflammation, which can cause disease and long-term tissue damage.

Important biological markers such as C-reactive protein (CRP)

One of the most crucial indicators for identifying inflammation in the body is C-reactive protein (CRP). CRP is a helpful marker for both acute and chronic inflammation since it is produced by the liver in response to inflammatory cytokines and its levels increase when inflammation occurs.

- **High-Sensitivity CRP (hs-CRP):** This test is very helpful in detecting silent inflammation since it may distinguish lower levels of CRP.
- **Elevated CRP Levels:** Low-grade chronic inflammation may be indicated by CRP levels greater than 1-3 mg/L.

- **Additional Markers:** Erythrocyte sedimentation rate (ESR), fibrinogen, and pro-inflammatory cytokines such as TNF-α and IL-6 are other indicators of inflammation.

By keeping an eye on these indicators, silent inflammation can be identified early and treated before it becomes a chronic condition.

2.2 Genetics' Function

Hereditary Propensities for Prolonged Inflammation
Because of differences in genes that control the immune system, certain people are genetically prone to chronic inflammation. These genetic differences may have an impact on:

- **Cytokine Production:** Excessive cytokine release may result from mutations.
- An extended period of inflammation may result from variations in the way immune cells react to stimuli.
- **Resolution of Inflammation:** The body's capacity to "turn off" the inflammatory response is compromised by certain genetic profiles.

For instance, certain variations in the TNF-α or IL-6 genes are associated with an increased risk of inflammatory conditions such type 2 diabetes, cardiovascular disease, and rheumatoid arthritis.

The Impact of Lifestyle on Gene Expression and Epigenetics.

Epigenetics is the study of how environmental and lifestyle influences, as opposed to changes in the DNA sequence itself, affect how genes are expressed. Genes linked to inflammation may be activated or silenced by these alterations.

The following lifestyle factors affect epigenetics:

- **Diet:** Diets high in fat and sugar can trigger genes that encourage inflammation.
- **Exercise:** Frequent exercise can reduce the expression of genes linked to inflammation.
- Prolonged stress has the ability to alter gene expression, which heightens inflammatory reactions.
- **Toxins in the Environment:** Gene activity that causes inflammation can be triggered by exposure to

chemicals or contaminants.

Knowing about epigenetics emphasizes how lifestyle decisions can reduce silent inflammation and stave off illness.

Acquired versus Inherited Inflammation Triggers"

Both genetic and acquired causes can cause silent inflammation:

- **Hereditary Triggers:** Among these are inherited genetic predispositions from previous generations. Silent inflammation is more likely to occur if there is a family history of autoimmune disorders or inflammatory problems.

- **Acquired triggers include:** These include lifestyle or environmental variables such stress, chronic infections, smoking, poor food, and inactivity.

Chronic inflammation is often determined by acquired stimuli, although hereditary factors lay the stage. The interaction of environment and genetics highlights the significance of leading a healthy lifestyle in order to reduce inherited risks.

2.3 The Effect of Inflammation on Organs

How Vital Organs Are Damaged by Inflammation

Over time, silent inflammation might impact several organs rather than just one. Persistent low-grade inflammation causes fibrosis, tissue damage, and decreased function. This is accomplished by:

- **Oxidative Stress:** Free radicals, which harm cells and tissues, are produced in greater quantities when there is inflammation.

- **Tissue Remodeling:** Prolonged inflammation may result in scarring or aberrant tissue development.

- **Impaired Blood Flow:** Inflammation can harm blood vessels, which lowers the amount of oxygen and nutrients that reach organs.

The following are examples that are specific to a particular organ:

1. Heart:

- Inflammatory cytokines can harm the artery lining, resulting in the development of plaque (atherosclerosis).

- The risk of heart attacks, strokes, and heart failure is increased by silent inflammation.

2. Liver:

- Fatty liver disease, fibrosis, and cirrhosis can all be brought on by chronic inflammation in the liver.
- Silent inflammation is closely associated with non-alcoholic fatty liver disease (NAFLD), which can lead to liver failure.

3. Brain:

- Alzheimer's disease, cognitive decline, and other neurodegenerative diseases are linked to inflammation in the brain.
- The blood-brain barrier may be broken by inflammatory cytokines, allowing dangerous chemicals to penetrate the brain's tissues.

Long-Term Effects of Untreated Inflammation If quiet inflammation is left untreated, there may be serious long-term effects:

- Type 2 diabetes, cardiovascular disease, arthritis, and neurodegenerative disorders are examples of chronic diseases.

- **Decreased Quality of Life:** Chronic pain, cognitive decline, and persistent exhaustion are prevalent.

- **Premature Aging:** Inflammation affects skin, organs, and general vigor by hastening cellular aging.

- **Increased Mortality:** Numerous diseases linked to inflammation, including cancer and heart disease, are among the world's top causes of mortality.

For management and prevention, it is essential to comprehend the science underlying silent inflammation. Our lives can be made healthier and less inflammatory by addressing biological mechanisms, hereditary factors, and organ-specific influences.

CHAPTER 3

Modern-Day Inflammation Triggers

3.1 Unhealthy Nutrition and Diet

The Connection Between Inflammation and Processed Foods

Processed and ultra-processed foods play a major role in modern diets. These foods tend to include a lot of harmful fats, processed sugars, and artificial additives, all of which can cause inflammation without being seen. Regularly consuming processed foods might cause your body's immune system to mistake them for dangerous invaders, which can result in a persistent inflammatory reaction.

There are several ways in which processed foods contribute to inflammation:

- **Preservatives and Additives:** Chemicals used to prolong shelf life might cause immunological reactions and disturb gut health.

- White bread, pastries, and sugary cereals are examples of foods that include refined carbohydrates, which raise blood sugar levels and trigger an inflammatory reaction.

- Processed foods are low in vitamins, minerals, and antioxidants, which means they don't provide the body with the nutrition it needs to combat inflammation.

Inflammatory Effects, Trans Fats, and Sugar

Trans fats and refined sugar are two of the strongest dietary causes of inflammation.

- **Sugar Refined:** Insulin and blood glucose levels rise when sugar intake is excessive. As a result, inflammatory cytokines including TNF-α and IL-6 may be produced in greater quantities. High sugar consumption over time leads to obesity, type 2 diabetes, and insulin resistance—all conditions associated with chronic inflammation.

- **Trans Fats:** Trans fats, which are present in baked goods, fried meals, and margarine, increase *low-density lipoprotein* (LDL) cholesterol while decreasing *high-density lipoprotein* (HDL) cholesterol, thereby contributing to inflammation. Heart disease is exacerbated by this imbalance, which destroys blood vessels.

The following must be reduced or avoided in order to lessen these effects:

- **Sugary beverages** such as sodas and energy drinks.
- **Fast food** that is heavy in sodium and trans fats.
- **Products with artificial sweeteners** that could interfere with intestinal health.

The Value of Diets That Reduce Inflammation

One of the best ways to fight silent inflammation is to follow an anti-inflammatory diet. Whole, nutrient-dense meals that lower inflammation and promote general health are the mainstay of this kind of diet. Important elements of a diet that reduces inflammation include:

- **Vegetables and Fruits:** Packed with fiber, polyphenols, and antioxidants (such as bell peppers, berries, and leafy greens).
- **Healthy Fats:** Omega-3 fatty acids, which are present in walnuts, flaxseeds, and fatty fish

(mackerel, salmon), help lower inflammation.

- **Whole Grains:** Fiber from quinoa, brown rice, and oats promotes intestinal health.

- **Herbs and Spices:** Natural anti-inflammatory chemicals can be found in garlic, ginger, and turmeric.

- Green tea is full of catechins, which have anti-inflammatory and antioxidant qualities.

An anti-inflammatory, well-balanced diet lowers the risk of chronic diseases, controls weight, and strengthens the immune system.

3.2 Environmental Aspects

The Contribution of Pollution to Systemic Inflammation
One major cause of silent inflammation is air pollution, a problem that permeates modern life. Particulate matter (PM2.5 and PM10), nitrogen dioxide (NO_2), and ozone (O_3) are examples of pollutants that can enter the lungs and cause inflammation and oxidative stress.

The following are important mechanisms by which

pollution causes inflammation:

- **Oxidative Stress:** Tiny particles enter the circulation and lungs, causing an excess of free radicals.

- Pollutant inhalation stimulates immunological cells, which in turn causes the release of inflammatory cytokines.

- The systemic effects include: Pollution-induced inflammation can impact the heart, brain, and other organs in addition to the lungs.

Pollution-induced inflammation has the following negative health effects:

- **Cardiovascular Disease:** Inflammation destroys blood arteries, raising the risk of heart attacks and hypertension.

- Pollution aggravates respiratory conditions like asthma and chronic obstructive pulmonary disease (COPD).

- **Neurodegenerative Diseases:** Dementia and cognitive loss may be exacerbated by prolonged exposure to pollutants.

Home Products' Chemicals and Their Impacts

Hazardous chemicals like phthalates, parabens, and volatile organic compounds (VOCs) are frequently found in common household products like air fresheners, cleaning supplies, and personal hygiene products. These substances have the ability to cause inflammation, irritate tissues, and interfere with hormone function.

Typical Inflammatory Chemical Sources:

- **Cleaning Products:** VOCs, bleach, and ammonia.

- **Personal Care Items:** Sulfates, preservatives, and synthetic perfumes.

- Bisphenol A, or BPA, is leaking into food and drink from plastic containers.

Select fragrance-free and eco-friendly products to lessen exposure.

For cleaning, use natural alternatives such as baking soda and vinegar.

Food should not be heated in plastic containers.

Risks of Radiation and Chronic Inflammation

Inflammation may be exacerbated by exposure to ionizing radiation (such as CT scans and X-rays) and non-ionizing radiation (such as cell phones and WiFi). Although modest doses of radiation are usually safe, excessive doses or prolonged exposure can cause inflammation and damage DNA.

- Ionizing radiation can lead to oxidative stress, cellular damage, and an increased risk of cancer.
- **Non-Ionizing Radiation:** Long-term exposure to electromagnetic fields (EMFs) may impair immune system function and sleep quality, although being less dangerous.

Limit needless medical imaging and lower EMF exposure by using hands-free devices and shutting off electronics at night to decrease dangers.

3.3 Stress and Lifestyle

The Inflammatory Reaction to Chronic Stress

One of the main causes of silent inflammation is ongoing stress. The hypothalamic-pituitary-adrenal (HPA) axis is triggered when the body experiences stress, which causes cortisol to be released. Prolonged stress upsets this equilibrium and increases inflammation, even if cortisol has an anti-inflammatory effect in acute circumstances.

Inflammatory Inflammation Mechanisms:

- **Increased Cytokines:** Stress causes inflammatory cytokines such as TNF-α, IL-1, and IL-6 to rise.
- **immunological System Dysregulation:** Extended stress maintains inflammatory pathways activated while impairing immunological defenses.
- **Impact on Gut Health:** Stress can alter the gut microbiota, which in turn causes inflammation via the gut-brain axis.

Mindfulness Practices

- Deep breathing and meditation are effective ways to manage stress.
- To control cortisol and release endorphins, engage in regular exercise.
- To boost immunity and lower inflammation, get enough sleep.

Disturbance in Circadian Rhythm and Sleep Deprivation

Sleep is necessary to keep the immune system in balance. Chronic inflammation and elevated inflammatory markers might result from sleep deprivation or circadian rhythm disruption.

Repercussions of Sleep Deprivation:

- **Increased CRP Levels:** A higher CRP and IL-6 level is associated with inadequate sleep.
- Lack of sleep has an impact on insulin sensitivity and metabolism, which increases the risk of obesity and diabetes.
- **Cognitive Decline:** Neuroinflammation is facilitated by poor sleep.

To enhance your quality of sleep, keep a regular sleep schedule.

Limit the amount of blue light you are exposed to before bed.

Establish a calming atmosphere that is chilly, quiet, and dark.

Sedentary Lifestyles as an Inflammatory Trigger

Silent inflammation is also mostly caused by physical

inactivity. Inactivity causes weight gain, lowers metabolism, and prolongs inflammatory processes.

The following are the mechanisms that connect sedentary lifestyles to inflammation:

- **Obesity:** Inflammatory cytokines are produced by excess fat tissue.
- **Muscle Atrophy:** Anti-inflammatory myokines are decreased as muscle mass is lost.
- Insufficient mobility hinders blood flow, which in turn fuels inflammation.

Remedies:

- At least 150 minutes of moderate exercise should be a weekly goal
- In order to preserve muscular mass, including strength training.
- By taking movement breaks throughout the day, you can prevent extended periods of sitting.

We may safeguard our long-term health by making educated changes if we comprehend how modern lifestyles, environmental circumstances, and bad food contribute to silent inflammation.

CHAPTER 4

CONDITIONS LINKED TO QUIET INFLAMMATION

Although it is not often obvious, silent inflammation is the cause of many chronic illnesses. Because of its sneaky character, it can progressively harm organs and tissues, which can lead to the emergence of severe medical disorders. This chapter examines the three main illness categories—autoimmune disorders, neurological diseases, and cardiovascular disease—that are associated with silent inflammation. We can find methods for management, prevention, and general health enhancement by comprehending these links.

4.1 Heart Conditions

How Plaque Buildup Is Caused by Inflammation

One important contributing factor to cardiovascular disease (CVD), the world's leading cause of mortality, is silent inflammation. Atherosclerosis, or the accumulation of fatty plaques in the arteries, is one of the main ways inflammation causes CVD. This is how the procedure goes:

1. **Endothelial Damage:** The endothelium lining of arteries may sustain damage due to inflammation. An inflammatory reaction is brought on by things like smoking, high blood pressure, and excessive cholesterol.

2. **Plaque Formation:** Inflammatory cytokines direct immune cells, especially monocytes, to the injury site. These cells develop into macrophages, which create foam cells by engulfing cholesterol particles. Fatty streaks that develop into plaques are produced by the buildup of foam cells.

3. **Plaque Instability:** The fibrous cap covering the plaque becomes weaker as inflammation continues. Plaque rupture is more likely as a result of this instability.

4. **Blood clots:** Blood clots can occur when a plaque ruptures, possibly obstructing the artery. This may result in a stroke or heart attack.

Associations Between Heart Attacks and Silent

Inflammation

One of the main factors that causes heart attacks is silent inflammation. An increased risk of cardiovascular events is linked to elevated levels of inflammatory markers such as interleukin-6 (IL-6) and C-reactive protein (CRP). Silent inflammation is a chronic condition that gradually damages blood vessels, in contrast to acute inflammation, which is a transient reaction.

The following are examples of chronic inflammatory triggers:

- **High LDL Cholesterol:** causes plaque to develop.
- Inflammation is fueled by insulin resistance, which is prevalent in type 2 diabetes.
- **Obesity:** TNF-α and other inflammatory cytokines are produced by adipose tissue.

Inflammation Reduction Techniques for Heart Health

Silent inflammation must be addressed in order to prevent and treat cardiovascular disease. Important tactics consist of:

Eating a Heart-Healthy Diet:

- **Mediterranean Diet:** Packed with whole grains, fruits, vegetables, omega-3-rich fish, and healthy fats like olive oil.
- **Reducing Processed Foods:** Cut back on processed carbs, sugar, and trans fats.

A minimum of 150 minutes per week of aerobic activity, such as swimming or brisk walking, is required for regular exercise.

Exercise for Strength: aids in lowering inflammatory indicators and increasing metabolism.

Management of Stress:

- Deep breathing, yoga, and meditation are some techniques that assist reduce inflammation by lowering cortisol levels.

Medications and Supplements:

- **Statins:** Provide anti-inflammatory and cholesterol-lowering effects.
- Fish oil contains omega-3 fatty acids, which lower CRP and other inflammatory indicators.

4.2 Disorders of Neurodegeneration

The Part Inflammation Plays in Parkinson's and Alzheimer's Disease

It is becoming more well acknowledged that silent inflammation has a role in neurodegenerative illnesses including Parkinson's and Alzheimer's. Inflammation speeds up the gradual loss of neurons that characterizes these disorders.

1. **Alzheimer's Disease:**
   - **Tau tangles and Amyloid Plaques:** Amyloid-beta and tau, two misfolded proteins, build up in the brain during Alzheimer's disease. More neuronal damage results from this accumulation because it causes the brain's immune cells, known as microglial cells, to release inflammatory cytokines.
   - **The Inflammatory Reaction:** Memory loss and cognitive decline are caused by persistent inflammation, which intensifies the degeneration of neurons.

2. Parkinson's Disease:

- **Dopaminergic Neuron Loss:** Parkinson's disease is caused by inflammation in the brain's substantia nigra, which damages neurons that produce dopamine.

- **Alpha-Synuclein Aggregation:** The misfolding of alpha-synuclein proteins, which results in Lewy bodies that hinder motor function, is encouraged by inflammatory processes.

Blood-Brain Barrier Inflammation-Related Breakdown

The blood-brain barrier (BBB) is a barrier that controls the flow of chemicals between the brain and the bloodstream. Silent inflammation can weaken the blood-brain barrier, allowing dangerous chemicals and immune cells to enter the brain and cause:

- **Increased Neuroinflammation:** Inflammation is exacerbated by immune cells invading the brain.

- **Oxidative Stress:** Free radicals accelerate neurodegeneration by causing damage to neurons.

- **Cognitive Impairment:** Neurological diseases and cognitive decline are exacerbated by disrupted BBB function.

Modifications to Lifestyle to Preserve the Brain

Take into account the following tactics to lessen the effects of silent inflammation on the brain:

Anti-Inflammatory Diet:

- **Nuts, berries, and leafy greens:** Packed with polyphenols and antioxidants.
- **Fatty Fish**: Omega-3s aid in lowering inflammation in the brain.

Workout:

- **Continuous Physical Activity:** increases BDNF, or brain-derived neurotrophic factor, which promotes the health of neurons.

Hygiene for Sleep:

- **7-8 Hours of Good Sleep:** vital for the lymphatic system's removal of brain poisons, such as amyloid-beta.

Mental Engagement:

- **Activities That Stimulate the Brain:** Learning new abilities, solving puzzles, and reading all support cognitive function.

4.3 Immune System Conditions

How Autoimmune Diseases Are Caused by Silent Inflammation

When the body's tissues are wrongly attacked by the immune system, autoimmune illnesses result. This process is greatly aided by silent inflammation, which produces a continuous state of immunological activation. Important mechanisms consist of:

- **Molecular Mimicry:** Because of their identical molecular structures, the immune system mistakenly believes that self-tissues are foreign invaders.
- **Dysregulated Cytokines**: Tissue damage results from the continuous production of inflammatory cytokines such as TNF-α and IL-17.
- Systemic inflammation and autoimmune can be triggered by dysbiosis, which is a disruption of the gut microbiome.

Common Conditions Like Rheumatoid Arthritis and Lupus

Silent inflammation is associated with a number of well-known autoimmune diseases:

- Systemic Lupus Erythematosus, or lupus, is a chronic illness in which the immune system targets several organs, including the heart, kidneys, and skin.
- Joint discomfort, exhaustion, rashes, and organ inflammation are examples of inflammatory symptoms.

An autoimmune condition that affects the joints and causes pain, swelling, and stiffness is called rheumatoid arthritis (RA).

- **Inflammatory Markers:** Rheumatoid factor (RF) and CRP are elevated.

Control Techniques to Lower Inflammation

Reducing inflammation and promoting immunological homeostasis are essential for the effective management of autoimmune disorders:

Dietary Adjustments:

- **Anti-Inflammatory Foods**: Include ginger, turmeric, fatty fish, and leafy greens.
- **Steer clear of triggers:** Steer clear of processed, dairy, and gluten-containing foods as they might make symptoms worse.

Regular exercise can help minimize joint pain and stiffness. Low-impact activities include yoga, swimming, and walking.

Mind-Body Practices:

- **Stress Reduction:** Deep breathing, awareness, and meditation all lessen inflammatory reactions.

Medications:

- **Immunosuppressants:** Assist in regulating hyperactive immunological reactions.
- **Biologics:** Focus on particular inflammatory cytokines (such as TNF inhibitors).

Knowing how quiet inflammation contributes to these illnesses emphasizes how crucial lifestyle changes and preventative interventions are. Early inflammation management can lower the incidence and severity of chronic illnesses, hence enhancing long-term health and wellbeing.

CHAPTER 5

SILENT INFLAMMATION DIAGNOSIS

Unlike acute inflammation, silent inflammation frequently goes unnoticed due to its subtle and sneaky signs. However, if ignored, it can lead to long-term illnesses such autoimmune diseases, neurological diseases, and cardiovascular issues. A comprehensive strategy that incorporates symptom awareness, focused laboratory testing, and a holistic perspective on health is necessary to diagnose silent inflammation. This chapter thoroughly examines various diagnostic options to assist you in recognizing and successfully treating silent inflammation.

5.1 Recognizing Signs

Quiet Indications of Inflammation

Under the radar, silent inflammation frequently takes the form of seemingly insignificant discomfort or general exhaustion. Silent inflammation has more subtle symptoms than acute inflammation, which has more overt manifestations like redness, swelling, or discomfort. Typical subliminal clues are as follows:

- **Persistent Fatigue**: Constant fatigue that doesn't go away when you take a break.

- **Brain Fog:** Mental sluggishness, forgetfulness, and difficulty focusing.

- Gas, bloating, and irregular bowel motions are examples of digestive issues.

- Acne, eczema, and inexplicable rashes are examples of skin problems.

- **Muscle and Joint Stiffness:** minor, inexplicable pains or stiffness in the morning.

Despite their apparent disconnection, these symptoms point to an underlying inflammatory condition when taken as a whole.

How Other Conditions Are Mimicked by Inflammation

The fact that silent inflammation's symptoms frequently coexist with those of other illnesses makes diagnosis difficult. For instance:

- **Brain fog and fatigue:** These symptoms are typical of depression, chronic fatigue syndrome, and thyroid diseases.

- The Digestive Issues: Food intolerances or irritable bowel syndrome (IBS) can be mistaken for silent inflammation.

- **Sore Joints:** This could be confused with musculoskeletal injuries or early-stage arthritis.

Due to these overlaps, people and medical professionals may fail to recognize the underlying cause of inflammation. This is why diagnosing unexplained symptoms requires taking a broad view.

Early Warning Indications to Look Out for

Early detection of silent inflammation can stop long-term harm. Keep an eye out for these warning indicators:

- **Inexplicable Weight Gain:** Particularly in the abdominal area.

- A weakened immune system as a result of persistent inflammation is the cause of frequent infections.

- **Sleep Disturbances:** Inadequate sleep or a sense of being unrested upon awakening.
- **Mood Shifts**: heightened irritation, anxiety, or depression.
- **High blood pressure:** An indication of inflammation in the arteries.

The development of diseases linked to inflammation can be stopped by identifying these early warning signs and pursuing prompt action.

5.2 Tests in the Lab

Important Tests, Such as CRP, ESR, and Others

Silent inflammation diagnosis requires laboratory tests. A combination of indicators can provide a more comprehensive picture, even though no one test can offer a conclusive diagnosis:

1. C-Reactive Protein (CRP):

- **What It Measures:** To combat inflammation, the liver produces CRP. Active inflammation is indicated by elevated CRP values.

- Lower than 1 mg/L is the normal range.
- The hs-CRP, or high sensitivity CRP, is more accurate in identifying low-grade inflammation associated with cardiovascular disease.

2. Erythrocyte Sedimentation Rate (ESR):

- The rate at which red blood cells settle in a tube over the course of an hour is what it measures. Inflammation is indicated by a higher rate.
- The normal range is usually between 0 and 20 mm/hr for men and between 0 and 30 mm/hr for women.

3. Levels of Fibrinogen:

- **What It Measures:** An increased level of the blood-clotting protein fibrinogen may be a sign of inflammation.

4. Role:

- **Homocysteine:** Inflammation and cardiovascular risk are linked to elevated homocysteine levels.

5. Inflammatory Insight:

- **Blood Glucose and Insulin Levels:** Increased insulin and glucose levels may indicate inflammation associated with metabolic dysfunction.

The Function of Imaging in the Identification of Inflammation

Imaging methods can be used to visualize tissue and organ inflammation in addition to blood tests:

- **Magnetic Resonance Imaging (MRI):** Good for identifying inflammation in soft tissues, joints, and the brain.
- Inflammation in tendons, ligaments, and organs such as the liver (such as fatty liver disease) can be detected by ultrasound.
- Positron Emission Tomography (PET) scans are useful for identifying systemic inflammation and inflammatory activity throughout the body.

In addition to test results, these imaging techniques aid in determining the location and degree of inflammation.

The significance of a thorough diagnosis

Silent inflammation is rarely diagnosed with a single test or symptom. A thorough diagnosis includes:

- Examining lifestyle, nutrition, stress levels, and previous medical issues is part of the detailed medical history.
- Examining mild and enduring symptoms over time is known as "symptom assessment."
- **Multiple Diagnostic Tests:** combining imaging, clinical assessments, and blood indicators.

This multifaceted strategy guarantees a more precise diagnosis and successful course of treatment.

5.3 The Value of a Holistic Approach to Health

Why Silent Inflammation May Go Unnoticed by Standard Tests

Conventional medical testing frequently focuses on identifying problems that are acute or evident. However, because silent inflammation is global and mild, it may go undetected by conventional diagnostic techniques. For instance:

- **Normal CRP Levels:** An hs-CRP test can identify low-grade inflammation that a normal CRP test might miss.

- Disregarding lifestyle factors: Comprehensive lifestyle evaluations are frequently left out of standard diagnoses, which leaves important inflammatory factors like stress or food unaccounted for.

For this reason, identifying hidden inflammation requires a comprehensive approach to health.

Combining Diagnostic Tests with Lifestyle Analysis

Lab results must be combined with a comprehensive lifestyle evaluation to diagnose silent inflammation. Important factors to think about are:

Dietary Habits:

- **Processed Foods, Sugar, and Trans Fats:** Evaluate the extent to which these factors influence everyday consumption.

- **Anti-Inflammatory Foods:** The existence or lack of

foods such as whole grains, veggies, and omega-3 fatty acids.

Chronic Stress Indicators:

- **Stress Levels:** Coping strategies, mental health, and work-life balance.
- **Stress Management Techniques**: Exercise, meditation, or neither.

Exercise Frequency and Intensity:

- **Physical Activity**: One factor contributing to inflammation is sedentary lifestyles.

Quality of Sleep:

- **Duration and Regularity of Sleep:** Inflammation can be exacerbated by inadequate sleep.

Collaborating with Medical Professionals to Deliver Proactive Care

In order to properly identify and treat silent inflammation, collaboration with medical professionals is essential. This proactive strategy consists of:

- **Collaborative Care Plans:** Including dietitians, physical therapists, and mental health specialists.

- **Regular Check-ups**: Arranged visits for tracking inflammatory indicators.

- **Patient Education:** By knowing how lifestyle decisions affect inflammation, people can take control of their health.

Integrative healthcare experts are better able to spot subtle patterns of inflammation and offer individualized, focused therapies.

Silent inflammation diagnosis is a complex process that calls for close attention to detail, extensive testing, and a full grasp of lifestyle factors. Silent inflammation can be identified and treated before it develops into chronic disease by identifying the mild signs, using focused diagnostic methods, and collaborating with skilled healthcare professionals.

CHAPTER 6

THE ANTI-INFLAMMATORY DIET.

Dietary Measures to Reduce Inflammation

A normal immunological reaction, inflammation can cause a variety of health problems, including obesity, autoimmune diseases, cardiovascular diseases, and neurological disorders, if it persists or becomes severe. The foods we eat are one of the most effective ways to fight silent inflammation. A carefully thought-out anti-inflammatory diet can avoid chronic diseases, improve general health, and drastically reduce inflammation. In-depth discussions of foods to stay away from, superfoods to eat, and useful meal planning techniques that support a low-inflammatory lifestyle are covered in this chapter.

6.1 Things Not to Eat

Typical Inflammatory Foods: Processed Foods, Sugar,

and Alcohol

It is well known that some foods cause the body to react inflammatory. Reducing or getting rid of these things is essential to preventing inflammation. The main offenders are:

Refined Sugars:
- **Sources:** Baked products, sodas, candies, sweetened cereals, and table sugar.
- **Impact:** Blood glucose levels are raised by refined sweets, which raises inflammatory indicators such as C-reactive protein (CRP). Consuming too much sugar also increases insulin resistance, which is a major cause of chronic inflammation.

Processed Foods:
- **Sources:** canned meals, packaged snacks, frozen dinners, and fast food.
- **Impact:** Typically, these foods contain high levels of sodium, trans fats, processed carbs, and artificial additives all of which exacerbate systemic inflammation. The body's inflammatory state is made worse by processed meals' deficiency in vital

nutrients.

Intoxication:

- **Effect:** Drinking too much alcohol affects liver function, raises inflammatory cytokine levels, and disturbs the intestinal microbiota. Over time, even moderate use might cause systemic inflammation.

Refined Grains:

- **Sources:** Pastries, pasta, and white bread are all produced using refined flour.
- **Impact:** Because refined grains are depleted of minerals and fiber, they raise blood sugar levels quickly and encourage inflammation.

The Role Allergens Play in Inflammation

Chronic inflammation may have a covert connection to food allergies. Inflammatory reactions can be triggered by intolerances or sensitivities even if you are not diagnosed with a specific allergy. Typical inflammatory allergens consist of:

- Rye, barley, and wheat all contain gluten. When they

consume gluten, those with celiac disease or gluten sensitivity have systemic inflammation.

- **Dairy:** Casein and lactose in dairy products can cause inflammation, especially in people who are sensitive to dairy or have lactose intolerance.

- **Soy:** Thyroid problems or sensitive people may experience irritation from soy products.

- **Oils Processed:** Omega-6 fatty acids, which are abundant in corn, soybean, and sunflower oils, can upset the ratios of omega-3 to omega-6 and cause inflammation if they are ingested in excess.

Identifying Dangerous Additives by Reading Labels

Learning to read food labels is essential to avoiding hidden inflammatory substances. Be mindful of:

- **Hidden Sugars:** Keep an eye out for words like dextrose, sucrose, glucose, and high fructose corn syrup.

- **Artificial Additives:** Steer clear of artificial coloring, flavor enhancers like MSG (monosodium glutamate), and preservatives like BHT (butylated hydroxytoluene).

- **Trans Fats:** Avoid partially hydrogenated oils since they have been shown to exacerbate inflammatory reactions.

You can take charge of your diet and reduce your inflammatory triggers by knowing what to avoid.

6.2 Superfoods That Reduce Inflammation

Avoiding unhealthy meals is only one aspect of an anti-inflammatory diet; another is adopting foods high in nutrients that reduce inflammation. You should incorporate the following potent superfoods into your diet:

Advantages of Green Tea, Ginger, Turmeric, and Omega-3s

Omega-3 Fatty Acids:

- **Sources:** Walnuts, flaxseeds, chia seeds, and fatty fish such as mackerel, sardines, and salmon.
- **Impact:** Omega-3 fatty acids aid in lowering pro-inflammatory cytokine and eicosanoid levels. They also promote joint mobility, brain function, and

heart health.

Curcumin (turmeric):

- **Impact:** Turmeric's main ingredient, curcumin, has strong anti-inflammatory and antioxidant qualities. Nuclear factor-kappa B (NF-κB), a crucial component of inflammatory pathways, can be inhibited by it.
- **Tip:** To increase the absorption of curcumin by up to 2000%, combine turmeric with piperine, or black pepper.

Impact:

- **Ginger:** Compounds found in ginger, such as gingerol, lower oxidative stress and inflammation. It works very well for reducing joint stiffness and muscular soreness.

Impact:

- **Green Tea:** Green tea, which is high in catechins like EGCG (Epigallocatechin Gallate), boosts immunity and lowers inflammation. Consuming it regularly can help fight chronic diseases and lower

CRP levels.

Inflammation Reduction with Fruits, Vegetables, and Whole Grains

Colorful fruits:

- **The following are examples of colorful fruits:** berries, cherries, oranges, apples, and grapes.
- **Advantages:** Rich in fiber, vitamins, and antioxidants. Fruit polyphenols fight inflammation and oxidative damage.

leafy greens:

- Swiss chard, spinach, kale, and arugula are examples of leafy greens.
- **Advantages:** abundant in the anti-inflammatory vitamins A, C, E, and K.... Additionally, they have magnesium, which lowers inflammation indicators.

Whole Grains:

- **Instances:** Barley, quinoa, brown rice, and oats.
- **Advantages:** Fiber from whole grains feeds good microorganisms in the gut, promoting gut health and

lowering inflammation.

Including Nutritious Fats and Oils

- **Avocados:** Packed with monounsaturated fats, avocados offer vital minerals like potassium and vitamin E while also reducing inflammation.
- **Olive Oil:** Rich in antioxidants, extra virgin olive oil contains oleocanthal, which has anti-inflammatory properties akin to those of ibuprofen.
- **Nuts and Seeds:** Good sources of fiber, antioxidants, and healthy fats include almonds, walnuts, flaxseeds, and chia seeds.

6.3 Organizing Meals to Reduce Inflammation

Useful Advice for Meal Planning

1. Batch Cooking:

- To make meal prep easier throughout the week, make big quantities of anti-inflammatory mainstays like quinoa, grilled salmon, and roasted veggies.

2. Use Herbs and Spices:

- To increase the anti-inflammatory properties of foods, add flavors such as turmeric, ginger, garlic, and rosemary.

3. Balance Your Plate:

- Try to have a plate that is well-balanced, including a range of vibrant veggies, lean proteins, and healthy fats.

4. Remain Hydrated:

- To aid in detoxing and lower inflammation, sip on lots of water and herbal teas.

Model Meal Plans to Reduce Inflammation

Breakfast:

- **Second Option:** Oatmeal topped with blueberries, chia seeds, and honey.
- **Second Option:** Avocado toast with a poached egg and a dash of turmeric on whole-grain bread.

The first option is grilled salmon served with quinoa and

steamed broccoli for lunch.

The second option is a mixed green salad with cherry tomatoes, walnuts, and a lemon-lemon dressing.

Supper:

- Secondary kale and sweet potatoes with roasted chicken.

- **Option 2:** Stir-fry brown rice, broccoli, bell peppers, and tofu.

The Value of Maintaining Dietary Routines

To reap the full advantages of an anti-inflammatory diet, consistency is essential. Adhering to these principles over time lowers the risk of chronic diseases and reduces systemic inflammation. Here are some pointers for staying consistent:

- **Plan Ahead:** Set aside time each week to prepare meals.

- **Maintain Healthful Snacks:** To steer clear of unhealthy selections, stock up on fruits, almonds, and hummus.

- **Mindful Eating:** To improve digestion, pay

attention to hunger signals and enjoy every bite.

You can actively fight silent inflammation and advance general health by avoiding inflammatory foods, adopting anti-inflammatory superfoods, and sticking to a planned diet plan.

CHAPTER 7

LIFESTYLE MODIFICATIONS TO COMBAT INFLAMMATION

Inflammation is a complicated process that is impacted by our everyday lifestyle choices in addition to our nutrition and genetic makeup. Stress, inactivity, and irregular sleep patterns can all make chronic inflammation worse. Thankfully, we may lower inflammation and enhance general health by making deliberate lifestyle changes. Three major lifestyle modification topics are covered in this chapter: stress reduction, physical activity, and sleep enhancement. When combined, these techniques provide a potent arsenal to reduce inflammation and promote long-term health.

7.1 Strategies for Stress Management

The Impact of Mindfulness and Meditation on Inflammation

One of the biggest causes of persistent inflammation is stress. Our bodies release cortisol and other stress hormones when we are under stress, and if these hormone levels are high for a long time, they can raise inflammatory markers like interleukins (IL-6) and C-reactive protein (CRP). Prolonged exposure to stress hormones can cause tissue damage, immune system suppression, and inflammation-related diseases such diabetes, autoimmune disorders, and cardiovascular disease.

Meditation:

To attain a level of calm, meditation calls for controlled breathing and concentrated attention. Regular meditation practice lowers cortisol levels and pro-inflammatory cytokines, according to studies. Methods that reduce inflammation-related biomarkers include guided imagery, mantra meditation, and body scan meditation.

Mindfulness:

Being completely present and conscious of one's thoughts, feelings, and physical sensations in the here and now is the practice of mindfulness. Programs for Mindfulness-Based Stress Reduction (MBSR) have been demonstrated to increase general wellbeing and decrease CRP levels. Practices that increase awareness and lessen the negative effects of stress on the body include mindful breathing, mindful walking, and mindful eating.

The Function of Counseling in Reducing Stress

For those who are struggling with chronic stress, anxiety, or trauma, therapy is a crucial part of stress management. Therapies such as Acceptance and Commitment Therapy (ACT) and Cognitive Behavioral Therapy (CBT) assist people in reframing negative thought patterns, creating coping strategies, and enhancing their emotional resilience.

The following are some advantages of inflammation therapy:

- It lessens anxiety and psychological suffering.
- Enhances emotional control, which lowers cortisol levels.
- Promotes healthy lifestyle choices like exercise and enough sleep that lower inflammation.

Exercise as a Stress-Relieving Activity

One of the best strategies to control stress and lower inflammation is to exercise. Endorphins are natural mood enhancers that are released by our body when we exercise. Additionally, exercise increases calm and reduces cortisol levels.

Suggested Activities:
- **Jogging or Walking:** A vigorous 30-minute stroll can dramatically lower stress hormones.
- A comprehensive method of stress reduction, yoga combines exercise, breath control, and mindfulness.
- Swimming is a full-body activity that reduces inflammation and encourages relaxation.

We can successfully lower inflammation and enhance general health by incorporating these stress-reduction strategies into our daily lives.

7.2 Exercises Power

The Direct Effect of Exercise on Inflammatory Markers

Systemic inflammation can be significantly reduced by engaging in regular physical activity. Exercise lowers levels of pro-inflammatory cytokines like TNF-alpha and IL-6 and increases the production of anti-inflammatory cytokines. In order to lessen inflammation associated with metabolic diseases, it also increases insulin sensitivity.

The mechanisms underlying the effects of exercise are as follows:

- **Muscle Contraction:** Exercise causes the production of myokines, which have anti-inflammatory qualities.

- **Improved Circulation:** Exercise improves blood flow, which helps tissues receive nutrients and oxygen while eliminating waste items that cause inflammation.

- **Weight Management:** By lowering adipose tissue, a major source of inflammatory cytokines, exercise helps maintain a healthy weight.

Yoga, resistance training, and aerobics are the best forms of exercise.

Different forms of physical activity are included in a balanced exercise program to optimize the anti-inflammatory effects. The best forms of exercise are broken down as follows:

Aerobic exercises:

- A few examples of aerobic exercises include swimming, cycling, running, and brisk walking.
- **Advantages:** boosts lung function, lowers CRP levels, and improves cardiovascular health.

Resistance training:

- Weightlifting, bodyweight exercises, and resistance band workouts are examples of resistance training.
- **Advantages:** lowers inflammation by improving insulin sensitivity, increasing muscle mass, and decreasing body fat.

Yoga and Flexibility Training:

- **Instances:** Pilates, Vinyasa, and Hatha yoga.
- **Advantages:** enhances flexibility and relaxation while lowering cortisol levels by combining movement and breath control.

Managing Intensity to Prevent Inflammation from Overtraining

Inflammation is decreased by regular exercise, but overtraining might have the opposite effect. Inflammation can result from excessive, high-intensity activity that is not sufficiently recovered from. This can raise cortisol levels and enhance oxidative stress.

Indications of Overtraining:
- Prolonged exhaustion
- Unresolved muscle discomfort
- Reduced performance
- Enhanced vulnerability to infections

Exercise Intensity Balancing Tips:
- Include active recovery sessions and rest days.
- Pay attention to your body and refrain from exerting yourself when you are too tired.
- Switch between low-intensity exercises like yoga or strolling and high-intensity workouts.

7.3 Circadian Rhythms and Sleep

The Importance of Restful Sleep in Lowering Inflammation

When it comes to managing inflammation, sleep is frequently disregarded. The body goes through vital processes of inflammation control, immunological regulation, and repair when you sleep. These mechanisms are disturbed by inadequate or poor sleep, which raises inflammatory markers like TNF-alpha, IL-6, and CRP.

Sleep Deprivation's Effect on Inflammation:
- Raises oxidative stress and cortisol levels.
- The body becomes more vulnerable to infections and long-term illnesses when the immune system is weakened.
- The equilibrium between pro-inflammatory and anti-inflammatory cytokines is upsetting.

Hygiene Advice for the Best Health

Inflammation can be decreased and sleep quality greatly enhanced by putting proper sleep hygiene routines into practice. The following are important tactics:

Maintain a regular routine by going to bed and waking up at the same time each day in order to control your circadian rhythm.

Sleep Environment:
- Make sure your bedroom is cold, quiet, and dark.
- Invest in pillows and a cozy mattress.

Set Screen Time Limits:
Avoid using electronics for at least an hour before bed in order to reduce exposure to blue light, which interferes with the generation of melatonin.

Relaxation Techniques:
- Before going to bed, engage in meditation or deep breathing.
- To help you relax, take a warm bath.

Melatonin and Other Natural Aids' Functions

- The pineal gland produces the hormone melatonin, which controls the cycles of sleep and wakefulness. It also possesses antioxidant and anti-inflammatory qualities.

Melatonin Supplements:

- Beneficial for people who have trouble sleeping because of jet lag, working shifts, or insomnia.
- **Dosage:** 30 minutes prior to bedtime, 0.5 to 5 mg are usually consumed.

Other Natural Sleep Aids:

- **Magnesium:** Promotes sound sleep by relaxing muscles.
- Apigenin, which is found in chamomile tea, promotes sleep and lowers anxiety.
- **Valerian Root:** Lowers sleep latency and improves sleep quality.

You may dramatically lower inflammation and enhance general well-being by practicing effective stress management, getting regular exercise, and placing a high priority on getting enough sleep. These lifestyle changes provide a strong basis for resilience against chronic illnesses and long-term health.

CHAPTER 8

THE ROLE OF SUPPLEMENTS IN REDUCING INFLAMMATION

Supplements are now a common weapon in the battle against persistent inflammation. By providing concentrated quantities of substances with anti-inflammatory qualities or completing nutritional gaps, they can support dietary and lifestyle changes. But it's important to comprehend their advantages, disadvantages, and role in a comprehensive health strategy. We will examine popular anti-inflammatory supplements, talk about possible dangers and adverse effects, and examine herbal therapies and traditional medicine in this chapter.

8.1 Typical Supplements to Reduce Inflammation

The potential of several substances to lower inflammation and promote general health has been thoroughly studied. Including these supplements can have specific advantages, especially for people with long-term inflammatory diseases.

Omega-3 Fatty Acids Among the most potent natural anti-inflammatory agents are omega-3 fatty acids, especially EPA (eicosapentaenoic acid) and DHA (docosahexaenoic acid). Omega-3 fatty acids, which are present in fish oil, flaxseed oil, and algae, aid in balancing the body's ratio of omega-6 to omega-3 fatty acids and lower the synthesis of inflammatory chemicals like prostaglandins and leukotrienes.

Advantages:
- Lowers CRP and other indicators of inflammation.
- Lowers blood pressure and lipids, which benefits heart health.
- Aids in the treatment of inflammatory diseases such as asthma, inflammatory bowel disease, and rheumatoid arthritis.

For overall health, aim for 1000-2000 mg of mixed EPA and DHA per day. Some inflammatory disorders may require higher doses.

Select premium, refined fish oil supplements to stay clear

of pollutants like mercury.

Vitamin D

Vitamin D is essential for controlling inflammation and the immune system. Increased inflammatory markers and an increased risk of autoimmune disorders are linked to a vitamin deficiency.

Advantages:

- Adjusts the immune system to stop overreactions to inflammation.
- Lowers the chance of developing long-term illnesses such diabetes, cardiovascular disease, and multiple sclerosis.
- Promotes bone health by facilitating the absorption of calcium.

The recommended daily dosage of vitamin D3 varies, although it is usually regarded as safe and effective at 1000-2000 IU.

- To find out if bigger dosages are required, have your blood levels checked.

Probiotics

Beneficial bacteria that support intestinal health are known as probiotics. Controlling inflammation requires a healthy gut microbiome because the gut contains 70% of the immune system.

Benefits:

- Decreases irritable bowel syndrome (IBS) symptoms and intestinal inflammation.

- Reduces systemic inflammation and boosts the immune system.

- Enhances the equilibrium of intestinal flora, lowering the proliferation of pathogenic microorganisms.

Dosage:

- Select probiotics that have at least 10-20 billion CFUs (colony-forming units) per dose and contain many strains (such as Lactobacillus and Bifidobacterium).

New Supplements: CBD Oil, Curcumin, and Resveratrol

As studies progress, a number of novel supplements have showed potential in the treatment of inflammation:

- Resveratrol is a polyphenol that can be found in berries, red wine, and grapes.
- By blocking NF-kB, a crucial inflammatory mechanism, it lowers inflammation and oxidative damage.
- The recommended dosage is 100-500 mg per day.

The main ingredient in turmeric, curcumin, has potent anti-inflammatory properties.

- **Benefits**: Inhibits cytokines and inflammatory enzymes (COX-2). aids in the treatment of metabolic syndrome, arthritis, and painful muscles.
- **Dosage:** 500-1000 mg daily with piperine (black pepper extract) for optimal absorption.

The hemp plant yields CBD Oil (Cannabidiol), which has analgesic and anti-inflammatory qualities.

- **Advantages:** Decreases anxiety, inflammation, and chronic pain. aids in the treatment of neuropathic pain and arthritis.

- **Dosage:** 20-50 mg daily; modify according to personal requirements.

Adequate Dosage and Purchasing for Efficiency

To guarantee efficacy and safety when utilizing supplements, quality and dosage are crucial:

Sourcing Advice:

- Select supplements from reliable companies that have undergone independent testing (such as NSF, USP, or ConsumerLab).
- Check for potency, purity, and the lack of impurities.

Consistency is Key:

- It frequently takes weeks or months of regular supplement use before any discernible effects are seen.

8.2 Hazards and Adverse Reactions

Supplements include hazards even though they can have a

lot of positive effects. It is crucial to use them sensibly and to be informed about any possible drug interactions or adverse effects.

Possible Contraindications to Medications

Prescription drugs and many supplements may interact, changing the medication's efficacy or producing negative side effects.

Common Interactions:

- **Omega-3s:** When combined with blood thinners such as warfarin, they may raise the risk of bleeding.
- **Vitamin D:** May have an impact on calcium levels and interact with cardiac medicines or diuretics.
- **Curcumin:** May conflict with diabetes drugs or anticoagulants.

Speak with a Healthcare Professional:

- To prevent harmful interactions, always let your healthcare professional know about any supplements you are taking.

Excessive Supplement Use and Its Effects

Supplement overuse can result in toxicity or other health problems:

Overuse Instances:

- **Vitamin D Toxicity:** May result in elevated calcium levels, renal damage, and cardiac problems.
- A compromised immune system or severe bleeding could result from an Omega-3 overdose.

Indications of Overuse:

- Headaches, exhaustion, nausea, or digestive problems.

Safe Supplementation Guidelines

Start Low and Go Slow:

Start with a lesser dose and increase it gradually according to how your body reacts.

Cycle Additions:

Do not take large amounts for an extended period of time

unless a healthcare provider advises you to.

To guarantee ideal dosages, test nutritional levels (such as vitamin D and omega-3 index) on a regular basis.

8.3 Traditional Medicine and Herbal Treatments

For millennia, people have tried herbal medicines and conventional medical procedures to treat inflammation. These techniques can be combined with contemporary medical care to provide a holistic approach to wellbeing.

Herbal Anti-Inflammatory Solutions' Advantages

Many active chemicals found in herbs have a synergistic effect of reducing inflammation:

Ginger:

- Lessens joint inflammation, stomach problems, and muscle soreness.
- Use: 500–1000 mg per day as supplements, dried, or fresh.

Boswellia (Indian Frankincense):

- Enhances joint function by inhibiting inflammatory enzymes.
- Standardized extracts (300–500 mg per day) are used.

EGCG, a potent antioxidant with anti-inflammatory qualities, is present in green tea.

- **Use:** 2–3 cups per day or 200–300 mg of standardized extracts.

Traditional Methods Such as Chinese Medicine and Ayurveda

Ayurveda:

- Balances body systems through the use of herbs, dietary changes, and lifestyle adjustments.
- For inflammation, try Turmeric, Ashwagandha, and Triphala.

Herbs, acupuncture, and nutritional treatment are the main tools used in Traditional Chinese Medicine (TCM), which aims to restore yin and yang equilibrium.

For instance, ginger, reishi mushrooms, and ginseng can help boost the immune system and reduce inflammation.

Combining Modern Healthcare with Traditional Remedies

A balanced strategy is provided by fusing contemporary medicine with traditional methods:

Insights for Integration:

- Collaborate with professionals who are knowledgeable in both conventional and alternative medicine.
- Verify that herbal medicines don't interfere with prescription drugs already in use.
- For optimal effects, combine evidence-based supplements with conventional methods.

When used as directed, supplements can significantly reduce inflammation. You may develop a comprehensive strategy that promotes long-term health by being aware of the advantages, dangers, and appropriate use of popular anti-inflammatory supplements and herbal therapies. To guarantee safety and efficacy, always get advice from medical professionals before beginning a new supplement regimen.

CHAPTER 9

NEW DEVELOPMENTS IN MEDICINE AND RESEARCH

Numerous diseases, including autoimmune disorders, cancer, and cardiovascular ailments, are largely influenced by chronic inflammation. New studies and therapeutic strategies are being developed as our knowledge of inflammation expands to provide improved options for treatment, early detection, and prevention. This chapter will examine the most recent developments in the study of inflammation, innovative therapies, and potential avenues for addressing chronic inflammation in the future.

9.1 Progress in the Knowledge of Inflammation

Inflammation is now recognized as a complicated and multifaceted process that underlies a wide range of chronic disorders, rather than only being a normal immune response to damage or infection. Cytokines, molecular pathways, and the identification of novel biomarkers for early detection are at the center of the most important advances in our understanding of inflammation.

Advances in Molecular and Cytokine Research

Immune cells create signaling proteins called cytokines, which are essential for controlling the inflammatory response. Studies on cytokines have shed important light on the causes of inflammation and its management. The identification of cytokine storms, in which an overabundance of cytokines results in extensive tissue destruction and is frequently seen in illnesses like COVID-19 and autoimmune disorders, is among the most encouraging discoveries.

Pro-inflammatory cytokines, such as TNF-alpha, IL-1, and IL-6, have been found to be important contributors to chronic inflammation. Many inflammatory disorders, such as rheumatoid arthritis, inflammatory bowel disease (IBD), and even some types of cancer, have high amounts of these substances.

On the other hand, cytokines such as IL-10 and

TGF-beta provide protective functions by preventing inflammation. There are now more opportunities for medicinal development thanks to research into improving these anti-inflammatory cytokines.

Targeting Specific Cytokine Pathways: TNF inhibitors and other biologics that target particular cytokine pathways have already transformed the way that conditions like Crohn's disease and rheumatoid arthritis are treated. The goal of ongoing research is to find even more targeted cytokine inhibitors that may be able to more precisely treat a wider variety of inflammatory diseases.

New Early Detection Biomarkers

The discovery of inflammatory biomarkers could completely change how chronic diseases are diagnosed and tracked. Measurable indications of a biological process or illness, biomarkers provide more focused treatment, improved prognosis, and earlier discovery.

C-Reactive Protein (CRP): CRP is a recognized indicator of inflammation in the system. Conditions like diabetes, inflammatory diseases, and heart disease are linked to elevated CRP levels. Ongoing research, however, aims to improve CRP testing so that it can identify inflammation early and enable earlier therapies.

Another promising marker is procalcitonin (PCT), which is particularly useful for differentiating between viral and bacterial infections. It may develop into a crucial marker for illnesses including sepsis and autoimmune diseases, although its function in chronic inflammatory states is still being investigated.

New Potential Biomarkers: metabolites and microRNAs are also being studied by researchers as possible biomarkers for chronic inflammation. These molecules may help identify those who are at risk even before symptoms appear, enabling even more accurate identification of diseases linked to inflammation.

Estimating Diseases Associated with Inflammation

Thanks to developments in genomics and personalized medicine, scientists can now use lifestyle evaluations and genetic profiling to predict an individual's risk of acquiring diseases linked to inflammation.

- **Genetic Risk Factors:** A higher risk of chronic diseases and an elevated inflammatory response are associated with specific gene variants. Variations in the IL-6 gene, for instance, have been linked to a higher risk of cardiovascular and autoimmune illnesses. Early intervention and customized preventative measures are made possible by the identification of these genetic markers.

- **Lifestyle and Environmental Factors:** Research is progressively demonstrating that a person's inflammatory response can be influenced by environmental pollutants, stress, and food. Researchers can create predictive models that assist in identifying people who might benefit from early anti-inflammatory therapies by having a better understanding of these aspects.

9.2 Innovative Therapies

New therapeutics that surpass traditional therapy are being developed as our understanding of inflammation advances. These consist of immunomodulation, precision medicine, biologics, and monoclonal antibodies.

Monoclonal antibodies and biologics

Large, intricate proteins called biologics are made to target particular components that contribute to inflammation. These treatments have revolutionized the way that inflammatory disorders, autoimmune diseases, and even some types of cancer are treated.

TNF-alpha Inhibitors: Drugs such as etanercept and infliximab block TNF-alpha, a major proinflammatory cytokine. Rheumatoid arthritis, ankylosing spondylitis, and IBD are among the ailments that these medications are used to treat. For patients suffering from chronic inflammatory illnesses, they have demonstrated efficacy in lowering inflammation and enhancing quality of life.

- **IL-6 Inhibitors:** Tocilizumab and other medications target IL-6, another important cytokine implicated in inflammation. In addition to being used to treat diseases including rheumatoid arthritis, these drugs are currently being researched for usage in cancer and COVID-19.

Autoimmune Disease Monoclonal Antibodies:

Targeting particular immune system components and stopping them from attacking the body's tissues is another promising use of monoclonal antibodies. For instance, Rituximab targets CD20 on B cells, which is a major factor in autoimmune illnesses such as rheumatoid arthritis and lupus.

The Function of Precision Medicine in Treating Inflammation

Based on lifestyle, environmental, and genetic factors, precision medicine customizes treatment for each patient. One important area where precision medicine has a lot of potential is inflammation.

- **Genomic Profiling:** Physicians can determine a person's genetic susceptibilities to diseases linked to inflammation by examining their genome. For instance, treatments that target IL-6 may be beneficial for people who have a genetic tendency to greater levels of this cytokine.

- **Personalized Drug Selection:** Using the patient's genetic profile, precision medicine also makes it possible to choose medications that have a higher chance of working. For example, a person's response to some anti-inflammatory medications may be influenced by genetic differences in drug-metabolizing enzymes.

Immunomodulation as a Prospect for the Future

One prospective avenue for the treatment of disorders linked to inflammation in the future is immunomodulation, which involves modifying the activity of the immune system. The goal of immunomodulation is to bring the immune system back into equilibrium rather than just reduce inflammation.

- **Immune Tolerance:** The goal of immune tolerance

research is to prevent autoimmune illnesses by teaching the immune system to identify and tolerate self-tissues. Tolerogenic vaccines are one possible strategy that could instruct the immune system to refrain from attacking its own cells.

- **Immune System Reprogramming**: Reprogramming immune cells to either increase their anti-inflammatory capabilities or decrease their pro-inflammatory reactions is another line of inquiry. This may result in better therapies for conditions like rheumatoid arthritis, multiple sclerosis, and Crohn's disease.

9.3 Looking to the Future

Looking ahead, a number of factors are influencing the study and treatment of inflammation. These trends center on increasingly individualized, efficient therapies as well as worldwide disease prevention measures related to inflammation.

Current Developments in the Study of Silent

focused treatments intended to lower inflammation before it results in long-term harm.

Public Health Preventive Strategies

A multifaceted strategy, involving lifestyle changes, public health campaigns, and improved access to healthcare, is needed to prevent chronic diseases linked to inflammation.

- **Encouraging Healthy Diets:** Public health initiatives that emphasize anti-inflammatory diets, such the Mediterranean diet or plant-based diets, can lessen the global burden of diseases linked to inflammation.

- **Reducing Environmental Toxins:** Lowering pollution and exposure to dangerous chemicals in the environment may also have a major impact on lowering chronic inflammation and the diseases that are linked to it.

International Initiatives to Address Inflammation-Related Chronic Illnesses

The importance of chronic inflammation to global health is becoming more widely acknowledged by institutions such as the World Health Organization (WHO). Coordinated efforts between governments, researchers, and healthcare systems will be necessary to combat chronic diseases like cancer, heart disease, and autoimmune disorders.

- **International Research Initiatives:** To better understand the processes of inflammation and create more potent treatments, international cooperation is crucial. In order to fight diseases linked to inflammation, these initiatives will concentrate on expanding access to treatments, carrying out extensive clinical trials, and exchanging knowledge.

Reducing the global health burden requires raising public awareness of the dangers of chronic inflammation and the significance of early detection and prevention.

People with chronic inflammatory illnesses now have new hope thanks to the quick advancements in inflammation research and treatment. We are beginning a new era of highly specialized, individualized treatments thanks to advances in cytokine research, the creation of biologics and monoclonal antibodies, and the expansion of precision medicine. Future developments will center on prevention, early detection, and international initiatives to fight inflammation and the diseases that are linked to it. As studies

keeps on, the possibility of better patient outcomes and quality of life will only increase.

CHAPTER 10

A Wholesome Strategy for Reversing Quiet

Inflammation

A mild but widespread ailment, silent inflammation can go undiagnosed for years and seriously harm the body. It frequently has a significant impact on the onset of long-term illnesses such diabetes, heart disease, arthritis, and neurological disorders. Fortunately, a thorough and individualized strategy can reverse silent inflammation. By implementing lifestyle modifications, creating a network of support, and guaranteeing long-term health, this chapter will present a strategic strategy to lessen and possibly even reverse silent inflammation.

10.1 Creating a Customized Anti-Inflammatory Strategy

A comprehensive, tailored strategy that incorporates nutrition, exercise, stress reduction, and customized therapies is the first step in reversing silent inflammation. It is feasible to lower inflammatory markers and enhance general health by implementing focused adjustments in these crucial areas.

Bringing Stress Management, Exercise, and Diet Together

Addressing the three main determinants of inflammation: diet, exercise, and stress is the cornerstone of any anti-inflammatory strategy.

Diet to Reduce Inflammation:

Your diet has a significant impact on how you manage inflammation. While avoiding processed foods, sugar, and trans fats, an anti-inflammatory diet usually places an emphasis on nutrient-dense, whole foods that are high in fiber, healthy fats, and antioxidants. Important components consist of:

- Omega-3 fatty acids, which are present in walnuts, flaxseeds, and fatty fish like salmon, sardines, and mackerel, help lower inflammation by regulating the synthesis of pro-inflammatory cytokines.

- **Vegetables and Fruits:** These foods, which are rich in vitamins, minerals, and antioxidants, aid in preventing oxidative stress, which fuels inflammation. Citrus fruits, berries, and cruciferous vegetables like Brussels sprouts, kale, and broccoli are very healthy.

- **Whole Grains and Fiber:** Foods such as lentils, brown rice, quinoa, and oats include fiber, which aids in blood sugar regulation and gut health, both of which are critical for reducing systemic inflammation.

- **Spices and Herbs:** You can reduce inflammation by including anti-inflammatory spices in your food, such as ginger, garlic, cinnamon, and turmeric (curcumin). It has been demonstrated that these herbs directly reduce inflammation by blocking pro-inflammatory enzymes and pathways.

- **Exercise:** One of the most effective strategies for

combating silent inflammation is regular exercise. Exercise lowers inflammatory cytokine levels, especially moderate-intensity exercises like yoga, cycling, swimming, and walking. Additionally, it encourages the release of myokines, which are anti-inflammatory chemicals made by muscle cells during exercise.

- Walking, running, and swimming are examples of aerobic exercises that improve cardiovascular health, lower visceral fat, which fuels inflammation, and promote general bodily functions.

- **Strength Training:** By increasing muscle mass, one can lessen chronic inflammation by increasing metabolism and decreasing body fat.

- In addition to enhancing posture and flexibility, yoga and stretching also assist lessen inflammation by promoting mental well-being and reducing stress.

- **Stress Management:** One of the main causes of silent inflammation is ongoing stress. Systemic inflammation results from the body's protracted release of stress hormones like cortisol, which also contributes to immune system dysfunction. Techniques for managing stress that work well include:

- **Mindfulness and Meditation**: Consistent mindfulness practices, such deep breathing techniques or meditation, can help the body relax and produce fewer stress chemicals.

- **Sleep Hygiene:** Reducing inflammation requires getting enough sleep. To help the body heal and boost immunity, try to get 7 to 9 hours of good sleep every night.

- **Time in Nature:** It has been demonstrated that spending time in green areas, whether it be for a stroll in a park or just being outside, lowers inflammation and stress levels.

Adapting Interventions to Specific Requirements

A customized anti-inflammatory regimen acknowledges that each person is unique and that their inflammatory response is influenced by a variety of genetic, environmental, and lifestyle factors. Interventions that are tailored may include:

- **Genetic Testing:** Knowing genetic susceptibilities to inflammation can help determine the best dietary modifications, supplements, or drugs to use.

- **Health Conditions and Medication:** It's crucial to think about certain dietary changes, exercise routines, and therapies that are in line with your condition if you currently have an inflammatory disease like lupus or rheumatoid arthritis.

- **Lifestyle Assessment:** A thorough analysis of lifestyle elements, including stress at work, sleep habits, and physical activity levels, can assist in identifying the areas that should be the focus of your anti-inflammatory strategy.

Monitoring Development Using Biomarkers and

Symptoms

Regular tracking is necessary to assess how well your anti-inflammatory plan is working. Important techniques consist of:

- **Blood Tests:** Regular testing for indicators of inflammation such as C-reactive protein (CRP), interleukin-6 (IL-6), and ferritin provide concrete proof of systemic inflammation reduction. Over time, a decline in these indicators suggests that your treatments are working.

- **Symptom Tracking:** You can monitor progress and make required plan modifications by recording symptoms like joint pain, exhaustion, and mood swings in a daily journal.

10.2 Establishing a Support Network

It takes more than one person to reverse silent inflammation. A strong support network can offer the motivation, information, and tools required for success.

Collaborating with Medical Experts

In order to help you navigate your anti-inflammatory journey, your healthcare team is essential. Important experts could be:

- **Primary Care Physician:** Your GP will assist in tracking your inflammatory indicators, evaluating your progress, and modifying your strategy as necessary.

- A registered dietician can offer customized dietary advice to make sure you're getting the nutrients you need while adhering to an anti-inflammatory diet.

- **Exercise Physiologist**: An exercise physiologist can design a safe and efficient program that encourages physical activity without overtaxing your body if you require a structured exercise program.

- **Mental Health Professionals:** Throughout your journey, a therapist or counselor can help you

Inflammation

Low-grade or silent inflammation frequently manifests without obvious symptoms, making early detection and treatment challenging. Nonetheless, it is believed that this kind of inflammation has a role in the emergence of numerous chronic illnesses, such as diabetes, heart disease, and neurological diseases.

- **Early Detection and Prevention:** Early detection of silent inflammation will become more possible as biomarker and molecular pathway research advances. The advancement of non-invasive diagnostic tools, such imaging or blood testing, will make it possible to identify those at risk for inflammatory chronic diseases early on.

- **Targeting Inflammation Before Symptoms Appear:** Future studies may concentrate on addressing inflammation early on to stop the development of chronic illnesses rather than waiting for symptoms to appear. This strategy might involve dietary adjustments, dietary supplements, and manage stress, deal with emotional triggers of inflammation, and support your mental health.

Including Friends and Family in the Trip

A strong motivation can be having a network of friends and family to lean on. By informing people of your objectives, they can:

- The ability of your loved ones to provide emotional support, hold you accountable, and acknowledge your accomplishments will help you stick to your strategy.

- **Participate Together:** You may create a good atmosphere where everyone gains from better habits by asking family and friends to join you in embracing an anti-inflammatory lifestyle.

- **Help with Challenges:** Family and friends can help out when things go tough, whether it's cooking or just lending a sympathetic ear.

The Function of In-Person and Online Support Groups

Online and in-person support groups can be excellent tools for meeting people who are traveling the same path. These organizations offer a venue for:

- **Sharing Experiences:** Gaining knowledge from others' triumphs and setbacks might make you feel less alone and offer insightful perspectives.

- **Access to Information:** Support groups frequently disseminate the most recent findings, inflammatory management advice, and therapy suggestions.

- **Building Community:** A sense of camaraderie that is fostered by group membership can offer the emotional support required to overcome obstacles.

10.3 Maintaining Health Over Time

Reducing inflammation and preserving long-term health are both essential for reversing silent inflammation. Sustainability necessitates ongoing attention to detail and adaptation.

Methods to Avoid Resuming Inflammatory Behaviors

Maintaining a healthy lifestyle is essential to preventing return when inflammation has been controlled. Among the tactics are:

- **Consistent Healthy Eating:** Include anti-inflammatory foods in your diet consistently, emphasizing nutrient-dense, whole meals over processed or inflammatory ones.

- **Maintaining Exercise Routines:** Continue your exercise routine to guarantee continued improvements in inflammation levels and general wellness.

- **Mindful Stress Management:** To control emotional triggers and avoid relapsing into high-stress states, keep up your mindfulness and stress-reduction practices.

The Value of Routine Examinations and Lifestyle Modifications

Make an appointment for routine check-ups with your healthcare team to guarantee ongoing improvement. These consultations provide chances to:

- **Monitor Biomarkers:** Monitoring inflammatory indicators on a frequent basis allows you to assess the success of your plan and determine what needs to be changed.

- **Modify Interventions:** Your strategy should alter as your health does. Maintaining the appropriateness and efficacy of your interventions requires regular reviews.

Marking Significant Progress in Reversing Inflammation

Reversing silent inflammation involves more than just curing illness; it also entails enhancing general health. Honor your accomplishments, no matter how minor:

- **Enhanced Vitality Levels:** Enhanced vitality and decreased exhaustion are potent markers of advancement.

- **Decreased Pain and Discomfort**: Less pain and stiffness is a big accomplishment for those with inflammatory diseases like arthritis.

- **Good Emotional Shifts**: The strategy is effective if there is a decrease in anxiety and depression, which are frequently associated with chronic inflammation.

Honoring these achievements gives you the drive to keep going forward and reaffirms your dedication to the goal.

The process of reversing silent inflammation is complex and calls for commitment, tolerance, and the correct support network. People can dramatically lower inflammation and enhance their general health by implementing a customized anti-inflammatory plan that consists of focused interventions, stress management, exercise, and food. Preventing relapse, adapting to life changes, and acknowledging accomplishments are all essential components of maintaining long-term health. Reversing silent inflammation is not only possible but also empowering when the proper resources and assistance are available.

ABOUT THE AUTHOR

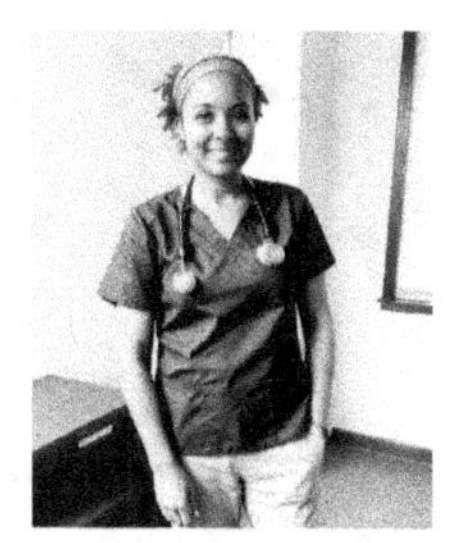 Harmony Royce is a dedicated healthcare worker who has a strong interest in holistic wellness. Harmony's extensive history in various aspects of health and wellness provides her with a wealth of knowledge and expertise that she can utilize in her writing and professional endeavors.

Harmony is a talented author who crafts thought-provoking books that inspire readers to have well-rounded, balanced lives. She writes about a variety of health-related topics, such as diet, exercise, mental health, and mindfulness. Her approachable writing style combines practical guidance with evidence-based research to make complex health concepts approachable and engaging for readers of all ages.

Harmony actively promotes the benefits of holistic health through writing, community workshops, and internet forums. Her mission is to educate and inspire people about the transformative power of self-care and healthy lifestyle choices.